Introduction by Richard F. Eisen,

It's a joy to see our children learning and growing. We teach them ... them hands. We teach them traffic safety and we teach them how to swim. ... these lessons help to keep them healthy and safe.

Skin cancer prevention and detection is another form of safety all children should learn at an early age. Skin cancers, including Melanoma - the most deadly form of the disease, are diagnosed in epidemic numbers in the United States, and are found in all age groups, including children. Fortunately, it is easy to help prevent this disease and, when it is detected early, it is almost always curable.

I urge you to teach your children five simple steps to help prevent and detect skin cancer. You can use the acronym, *SunAWARE,* as a daily reminder of what to do.

A – Avoid unprotected UV exposure at any time and seek shade.
W – Wear sun protective clothing including hats and sunglasses.
A – Apply sunscreen with an SPF 30+ prior to UV exposure and reapply every two hours while exposed.
R – Routinely check your whole body for changes in your skin and report new or changing skin growths to a health care provider.
E – Educate your family and community about sun protection.

This wonderfully illustrated book supports the 'R' of *SunAWARE.* It helps to teach young children about their skin – their moles and freckles. It uses and illustrates lessons from the American Academy of Dermatology and is a valuable tool for parents who understand that skin safety will help give children a healthy future.

Richard Eisen, MD
Medical Director - Children's Melanoma Prevention Foundation
Dermatologist at South Shore Skin Center, Plymouth, MA

SunAWARE has been endorsed by the Dermatology Nurses Association, the Children's Melanoma Prevention Foundation and Coolibar. The acronym was created for *Sun Protection For Life: Your Guide To A Lifetime Of Healthy And Beautiful Skin* by Mary Mills Barrow and John F. Barrow, which won a Gold Triangle Award for excellence in public education of dermatologic issues.

What Are These Spots On My Skin?

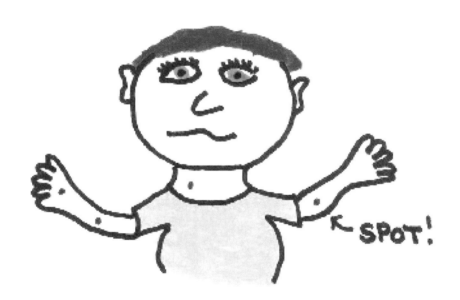

SPOT!

Written By Scott Naughton

Illustrated By
Gus Naughton and Scott Naughton

First published by AuthorHouse 2/28/2008

ISBN: 1-4259-0601-X (sc)

Printed in the United States of America
Bloomington, Indiana

This book is printed on acid-free paper.

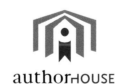

authorHOUSE

1663 LIBERTY DRIVE
BLOOMINGTON, INDIANA 47403
(800) 839-8640
www.authorhouse.com

I have spots
on my skin.

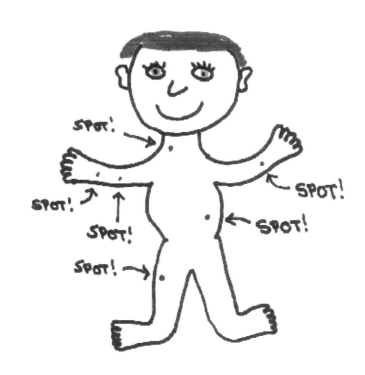

Can you find the letter "a"?
How many spots do you see on me?

Some are very dark.

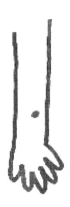

Some are kind of brown.

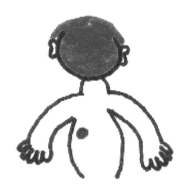

Some look red.

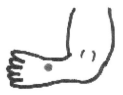

Can you find the letter "b"?
What other colors can you name?

Some are big. (Some have hair growing out of them!)

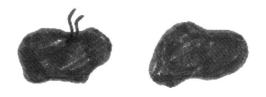

I can see some
small ones.

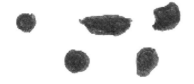

Some are medium sized.

Can you find the letter "c"?
Can you count the spots by each sentence?

I have a couple
that feel bumpy.

BUMPY
SPOT!

And some that
are so flat I can
hardly feel them.

FLAT
SPOT!

Can you find the letter "d"?
What does "bumpy" mean?

Some spots are
    called freckles.

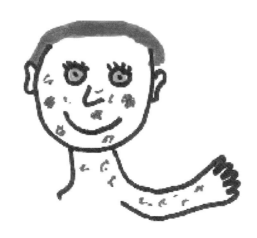

Some people call these spots
    "beauty marks".

I like that name best!

Can you find the letter "e"?
Can you find a spot on your body?

I have spots
on my arms.

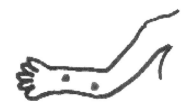

And four spots on
my belly.

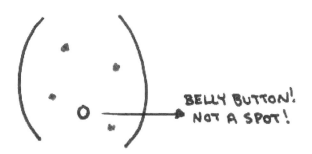

BELLY BUTTON!
NOT A SPOT!

Can you find the letter "f"?
How many spots do you see on my arm?

And some on my legs.

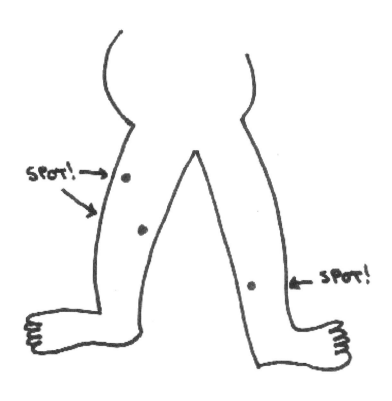

Can you find the letter "g"?
How many spots are on each leg?

There is a spot
between my fingers.

—SPOT!

And one between
my toes.

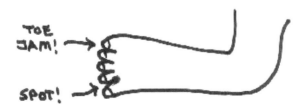

TOE
JAM! →

SPOT! →

Can you find the letter "h"?
How many toes do I have?

I wonder if I have some spots in places
  I can't see by myself.

Like on my back.

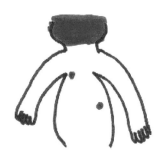

Or under
    my hair.

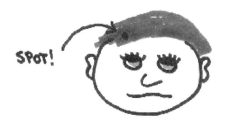

Can you find the letter "I"?
Are there other places on your body you can't see?

I'm just checking
behind my ears.

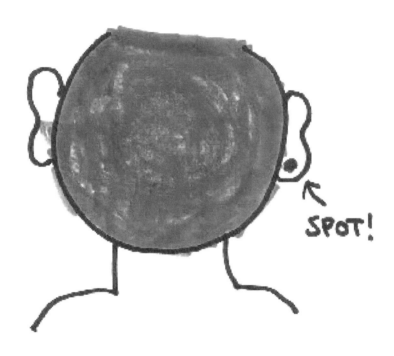

SPOT!

Can you find the letter "j"?
What color is my hair?

My Mommy or Daddy
or Aunt or Grandma
can look at those
places I can't see.

They know where
all my spots are.

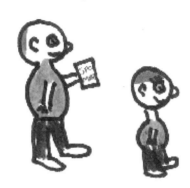

They keep track of
them on a spot map
of my body.

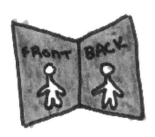

Can you find the letter "K"?
Who looks at your spots for you?

Where else might you find spots on your body?

Fingernails.

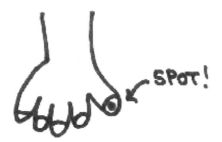

Toenails.

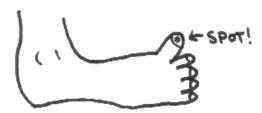

Can you find the letter "l"?
How many toenails do I have?

Are there any other
places I might forget
to look at?

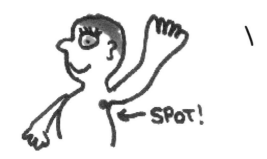

My armpits.

The bottom of my feet.

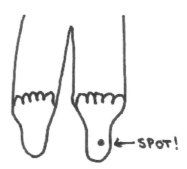

Can you find the letter "m"?
How many feet do I have?

Does everyone have
spots on their skin?

I see some on Mommy.

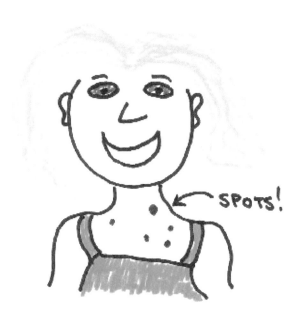

SPOTS!

Can you find the letter "n"?
How many spots does Mommy have?

I see some on
    Daddy, too!

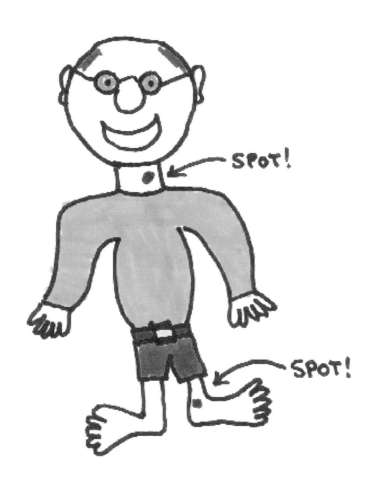

SPOT!

SPOT!

Can you find the letter "o"?
How many spots do you see on Daddy?

I wonder if Mommy and Daddy count the spots on each other. They probably do.

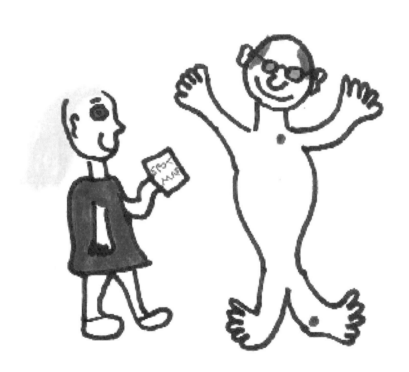

Can you find the letter "p"?
Does your family look at the spots on each other?

I have a question.

What are these spots, anyway?

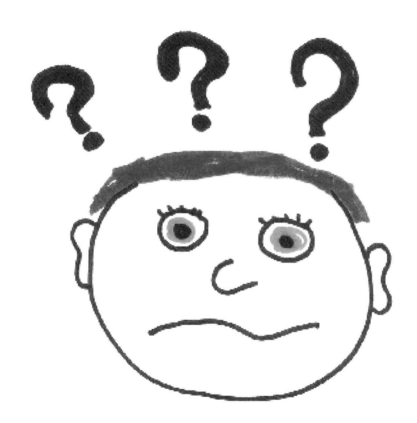

Can you find the letter "q"?
Can you find six question marks on this page?

Where do they
come from?

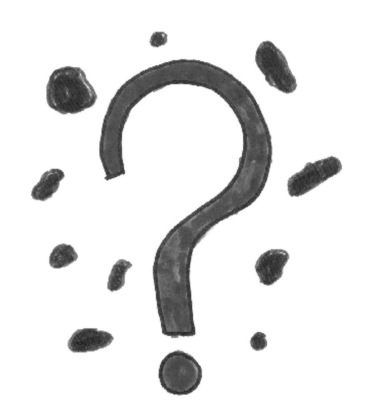

Can you find the letter "r"?
Where do you think these spots come from?

I guess they are a part of
my skin, but different.

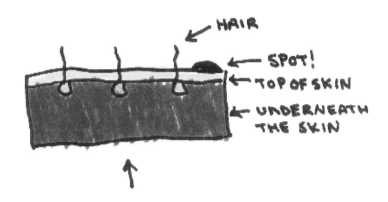

That is what my
skin would look
like under a
microscope.

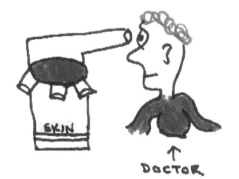

Can you find the letter "s"?
What is a microscope?

Here is a spot map of my body. I put a dot where
I have a spot, using a pencil or pen.
Hey, that rhymes...dot and spot!

front of me
(This doesn't really look like me.....)

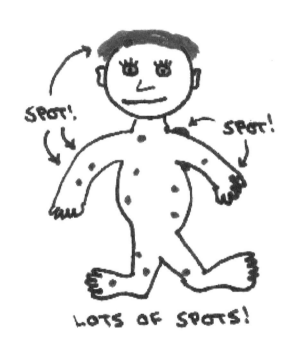

Can you find the letter "t"?
How many spots do you see on the front of me?

That way I can keep track of the spots on my skin. There is a spot map for you at the end of this book.

<u>back of me</u>
(....but I can use it anyway!)

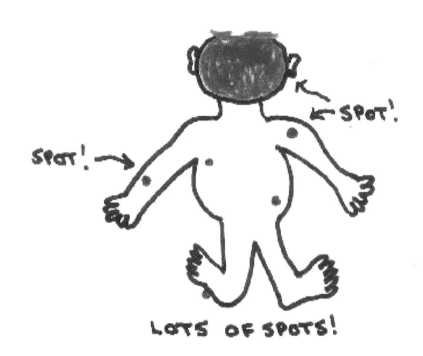

spot! →

← spot!

Lots of spots!

Can you find the letter "u"?
How many spots do I have on the back of me?

I check for spots on my
skin every year, right
around my birthday.

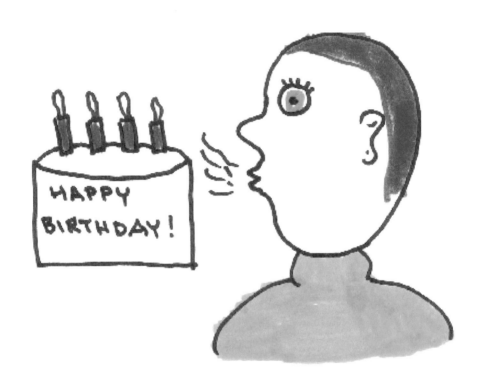

Can you find the letter "V"?
How many candles are on the cake?

Then I can see if I have new spots this year. I also can see if any old spots are different than they were last year.

last year   this year

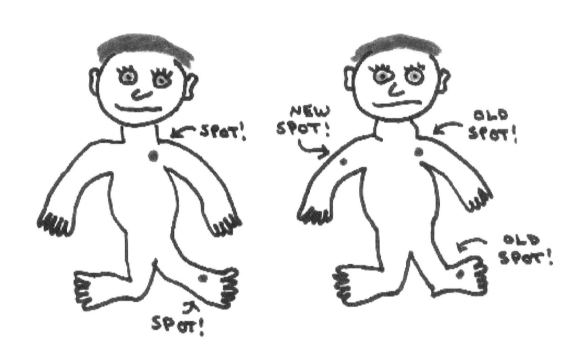

Can you find the letter "w"?
Do I have more spots this year than last year?

How can I tell if they
   are different?
What do I look for?
Do I need an x-ray?

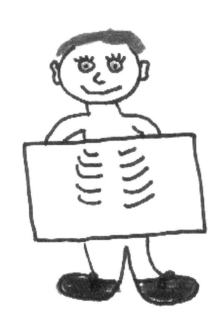

Nope!
All you need
is your eyes!

Can you find the letter "x"?
How many ribs do I have?

It's so easy!

I just look for

A, B, C, D

and
sometimes

E

Zoiks! Those are letters from the alphabet!

Can you find the letters "y" and "z"?

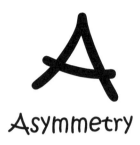

Asymmetry

That's a big word!

But all it really means is that one side of the spot is different from the other side of the spot.

asymmetrical   symmetrical

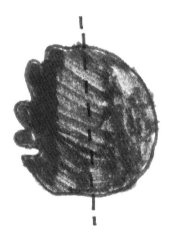   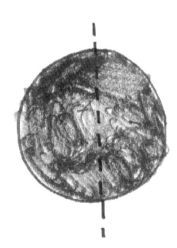

B

Border Irregularity

This is when the outside of the spot is not the same all the way around.

irregular

regular

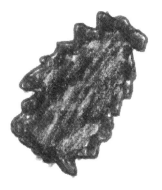

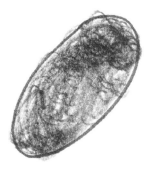

C

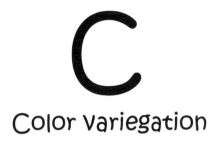

Color variegation

Are there different colors within the same spot, or has the color changed from last year?

different colors   same color

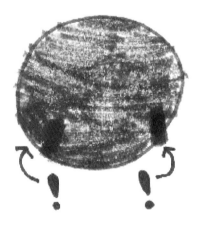

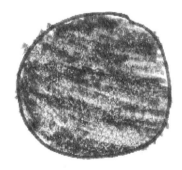

D

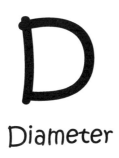

Diameter

Is the spot bigger than it was
last year, or is it a big, new spot?

last year   this year

                    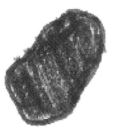

E

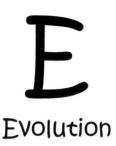

Evolution

Does the spot feel higher than it used to, is it starting to itch, or is it somehow different now than it used to be?

last year   this year

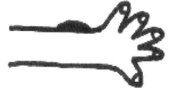   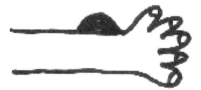

I put the map of my body
on the wall next to my
growth chart to remind
me to check my spots.

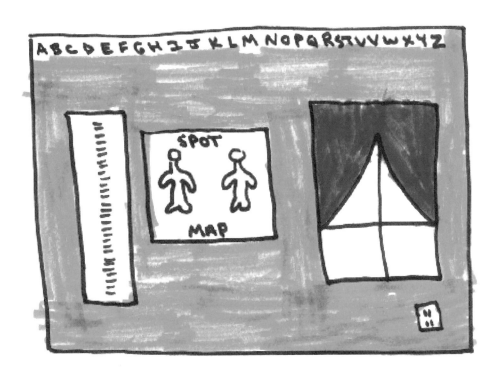

Your doctor knows a lot about the spots on your skin.

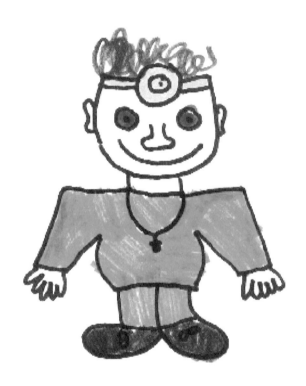

The next time you visit your doctor, ask him or her to look at your spots. See if your doctor can count them! Show the doctor the spot map of your body!

I think it's fun to keep
  track of my spots with dots!

(There's that rhyme again!)

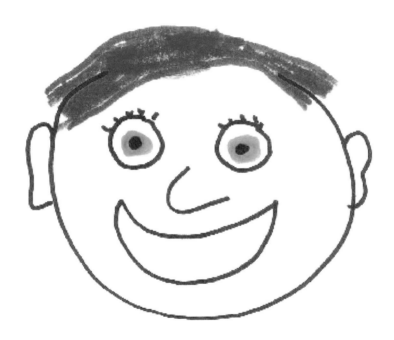

Try it!

Spot Map for (your name) _____

FRONT

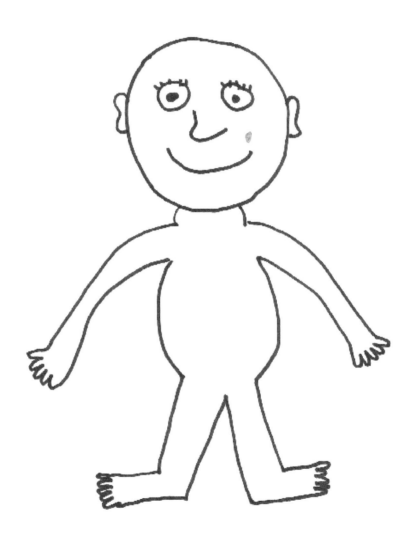

Spot Map for (your name) _____

BACK

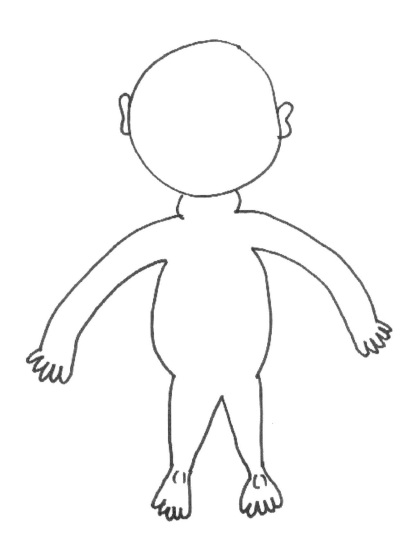

Extra Spot Map for (name)_____

FRONT

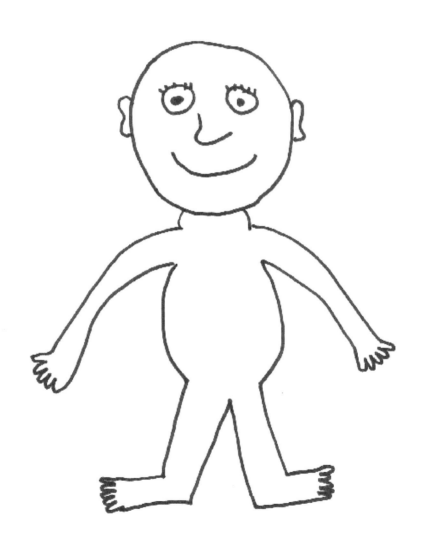

Extra Spot Map for (name)_____

BACK

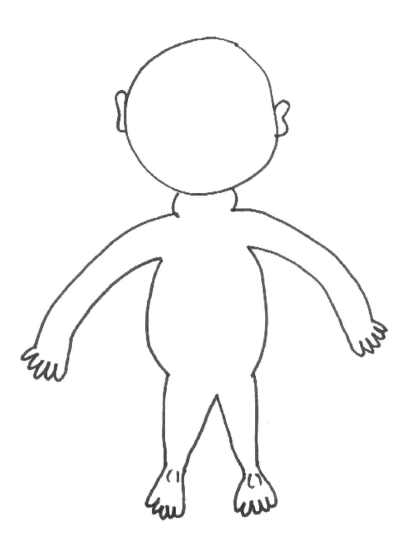

Printed in the United States
105866LV00002B